Ketogenic Recipes:

Nutritious, Delicious And Simple Ketogenic Recipes To Spike Your Metabolism And Burn Stubborn Fat

Kennedy Ross

Table of Contents

Introduction

Congratulations on purchasing your personal copy of *Ketogenic Recipes: Nutritious, Delicious And Simple Ketogenic Recipes To Spike Your Metabolism And Burn Stubborn Fat.* Thank you for doing so.

You are about to view many tasty recipes to enjoy while you experience your ketogenic diet plan. The low-carbs will cause ketones to be produced by the liver which will shift your body towards fat utilization. Not only is the plan a proven weight loss tool, but it is also shown to improve several health conditions including epilepsy, Parkinson's, and Alzheimer's.

You will discover how simple the approach is to a low-carb diet that is popular because you are consuming natural/real food products that are not full of preservatives and other additives.

There are many different ways to enjoy your breakfast as well as how to prepare beef, pork, chicken, duck, and seafood. Several salads and sides are provided for additional variations to your regular meals. A few low-carb desserts are shown so your 'sweet tooth' can also remain happy!

There are plenty of books on this subject on the market, thanks again for choosing this one. Every effort was made to ensure it is full of as much useful information as possible. Please enjoy!

Chapter 1: Breakfast Delights

Deviled Eggs

Ingredients
6 large eggs
¼ teaspoon yellow mustard
1 tablespoon mayonnaise
1 teaspoon paprika
Garnish: Parsley/salt/pepper
Optional:
- ½ teaspoon cayenne pepper
- Several drops hot sauce
- 1 teaspoon cumin

Instructions
1. Slice the eggs lengthwise.
2. Mix the egg yolks with the rest of the ingredients.
3. Stuff the eggs. Sprinkle with condiments as desired.

Carbs: 1.0 g each (serving of ½ egg)

Fisherman's Eggs

Ingredients
2 eggs
1 can of sardines
¼ onion minced
½ cup arugula
2 ½ tablespoons marinated artichoke hearts (TJ's is good)
Fresh black pepper
Pinch of sea salt

Instructions
1. Set the oven temperature to 375°F.
2. Flake the sardines and mix with the onion into a stoneware baking dish. Layer the broken eggs, arugula, with the artichokes as the top later.
3. Sprinkle with the pepper and salt. Bake for ten minutes until done.

Carbs: 3.5 g (one serving)

Fried Eggs with Pork and Kale

Ingredients
½ pound kale
3 ½ ounces butter
4 eggs
½ pound bacon or smoked pork belly
¼ cup frozen cranberries
1-ounce walnuts or pecans
To Taste: Pepper and salt

Instructions
1. Prewash, trim and chop the kale into large squares.
2. Melt the butter in a skillet and quick fry the kale on high heat until the edges are slightly brown. Transfer the kale to a container.
3. Sear the bacon in the same pan. Lower the heat and add the kale, nuts, and cranberries. Stir until heated and reserve in a separate container.
4. Fry the eggs with the remainder of the butter, and add a pinch of pepper and salt if desired.

Carbs: 10.0 g each (two servings recipe)

Frittata with Cheese and Tomatoes

Ingredients
6 eggs
2/3 cup soft cheese (ex. Feta 3 ½ ounces)
½ medium (1.9 ounces) white onion
2/3 cup halved cherry tomatoes
2 tablespoons chopped herbs (ex. basil or chives)
1 tablespoon ghee/butter

Instructions
1. Program the oven broiler to 400°F.
2. Place the onions on a greased, hot iron skillet and cook with ghee/butter until slightly brown.
3. In a separate dish, crack the eggs and add the salt, pepper, or add herbs if you wish. Whisk and add to the onion pan. Cook until the edges begin to cook.
4. Top with the cheese and tomatoes. Put the pan in the broiler for five to seven minutes or until done.

Carbs: 6.2 grams each (two servings in recipe)

Italian Egg Bake

Ingredients
10 large eggs
3 tablespoons mustard
½ cup heavy whipping cream
2 teaspoons garlic and herb seasoning
½ cup tomato sauce
2 cups chicken breast (cooked – diced)
1 (12 ounces) package frozen broccoli florets
½ cup grated Parmesan cheese
1 teaspoon parsley flakes
Optional: 1 cup shredded extra sharp cheese

Instructions
1. Preheat the oven to 350°F.
2. Whisk the eggs in a mixing container, and add the seasoning, mustard, and whipping cream. Whisk in the tomato sauce, stir, and add the chicken and florets.
3. Add to a baking dish and sprinkle the Parmesan cheese and parsley on the top and bake for 30 to 40 minutes.

Carbs: 4.38 g each (8 servings)

Mock 'Mc Griddle' Casserole

Ingredients
1 pound breakfast sausage
¼ cup flaxseed meal
1 cup almond flour
10 large eggs
6 tablespoons maple syrup
4 ounces cheese
4 tablespoons butter
¼ teaspoon sage
½ teaspoon each: onion & garlic powder

Instructions
1. Heat the oven in advance to 350°F.
2. Use medium heat and begin cooking the breakfast sausage on the stove in a skillet.
3. Blend all of the dry (the cheese also) ingredients and add the wet ones.
4. Add four tablespoons of the syrup and blend well.
5. After the sausage is crispy brown—mix all of the ingredients along with the fat.
6. Use parchment paper to line a 9 x 9-inch casserole dish.
7. Pour the mix into the baking dish and drizzle the remainder of the syrup on the top. Bake for 45 to 55 minutes. Let it cool.

Tip: The casserole should be easy to remove by using the edge of the parchment paper.

Carbs: 2.9 g each serving (recipe is eight servings)

Omelet Wrap with Avocado & Salmon

Ingredients
3 large eggs
½ package smoked salmon (1.8 ounces)
½ of an average sized avocado (3.5 ounces)
1 spring onion (1/2 ounce)
2 tablespoons cream cheese (full-fat—2.3 ounces)
2 tablespoons chives (freshly chopped)
1 tablespoon butter or ghee

Instructions
1. In a mixing bowl—add a pinch of pepper and salt along with the eggs. Use a fork or whisk—mixing them well.
2. Blend the chives and cream cheese.
3. Prepare the salmon and avocado (peel and slice).
4. In a skillet, add the butter/ghee, and the egg mixture. Cook until fluffy and soft.
5. Place the omelet on a serving dish, and spoon the mixture of cheese over it.
6. Sprinkle the onion, prepared avocado, and salmon into the wrap. Close and enjoy!

Carbs: 5.8 g each (2 servings)

Sausage Patties

Ingredients
1 teaspoon maple extract
2 tablespoons granular Swerve Sweetener
½ teaspoon pepper
1 pound ground pork
2 tablespoons sage (chopped fresh)
1/8 teaspoon cayenne
1 teaspoon salt
¼ teaspoon garlic powder

Instructions
1. Combine each of the ingredients in a large container.
2. Form the patties to approximately one-inch thickness.
3. Add a bit of olive oil or a dab of butter to a pan over medium heat.
4. For each side, allow three to four minutes cooking time.

Carbs: 1.4 g each (recipe for 2 patties)

Sausage—Feta—Spinach Omelet

Ingredients
½ tablespoon extra-virgin olive oil
2 sausage links
3 large eggs
¼ cup Half & Half
1 cup spinach
1 tablespoon feta cheese

Instructions
1. You will need two skillets. Use medium heat for both pans, and pour olive oil in one of the two.
2. In a small dish, use the Half & Half and mix with the eggs—add the seasonings—and scramble.
3. In the clean pan, cook the sausage.
4. Sauté the spinach in the oiled pan—add a bit of salt and pepper if desired.
5. After both have finished cooking, combine them in a bowl.
6. Transfer the olive oiled pan to the sausage fat pan—and add the eggs.
7. When the edges begin to cook—add the spinach, sausage, and cheese.
8. Cook another minute—flip the omelet. Cook another two to three minutes.
9. Cover one pan with the other and let the combo steam.
10. Remove and enjoy!

Carbs: 3 g (1 serving recipe)

Scrambled Eggs and Bacon

Ingredients for the Eggs:
3 large eggs
Fresh ground pepper
Coarse salt
1 tablespoon unsalted butter

Instructions for the Eggs:
1. Whisk the eggs in a bowl.
2. Use low heat and place the butter in a skillet. Add the eggs.
3. Continue to stir until well-done, usually 1 ½ to 3 minutes.

Carbs: 1.8 g (1 serving recipe)

How to Prepare the Bacon:

Use the Regular Oven:
1. Preheat to 350 °F. Place the bacon on a baking tray and bake 20 to 25 minutes
2. Drain on a paper towel.

Use the Microwave:
1. Put the bacon on paper towels in a single layer on a microwave-safe dish.
2. Use the high setting for four to six minutes.

Use the Skillet:
1. Prepare the pan on medium-low to medium. Arrange the bacon in the pan single-layered.
2. Cook until the desired doneness is acquired.

Carbs: 0.0 g (2 slices)

Sesame Buns

Ingredients
½ cup pumpkin seeds
½ cup sesame seeds (+) ½ cup to cover the buns
1 cup coconut flour
½ cup psyllium powder
1 tablespoon sea salt
8 egg whites
1 cup hot water
1 tablespoon baking powder

Instructions
1. Set the oven to 350°F.
2. Mix the dry ingredients. Blend the egg whites in a blender until foamy.
3. Combine them (#2) in a food processor until crumbly.
4. Add one cup boiling water and stir to create a smoother dough. Make 12 buns.
5. Empty the additional ½ cup sesame seeds in a dish and cover the top side of the bun. Arrange the buns on a parchment paper covered cookie sheet. Bake for 50 minutes.
6. For a crunchy top, let the buns cool down in the oven.

Carbs: 4.0 g each (12 buns in the recipe)

Shakshuka

Ingredients
1 can crushed tomatoes (San Marzano)
¼ cup olive oil
½ small – finely diced - yellow onion
2 garlic cloves
Pinch of red pepper flakes
1 bay leaf (optional)
½ teaspoon each:
- Cumin
- Paprika
- Cayenne

1 teaspoon each:
- Pepper
- Salt
- Garlic powder

4 fresh eggs
Garnishes:
- Crumbled feta cheese
- 4 tablespoons chopped basil

Instructions
1. Warm the oil in a skillet using medium heat. Toss in the garlic and onions and sauté for a couple of minutes. Add the tomatoes, herbs (omit basil), and spices.
2. Reduce the heat and simmer about 30 minutes. Crack the eggs on the top of the sauce. Cover and allow the steam to work until the eggs are firm for about three to four minutes.
3. Top it off with some pepper, salt, basil, and feta cheese if you wish.

Carbs: 4.8 g each (4 servings)

Spinach Alfredo & Avocado Eggs

Ingredients
1 (5 ounces) bag spinach
1 (22 ounces) bottle garlic Alfredo sauce
6 eggs
Pepper and salt
Optional: ½ avocado

Instructions
1. Use high heat and simmer the sauce. Toss in the spinach and cook about one to two minutes until it wilts.
2. Make six sections in the mixture and add the eggs. Cook about five to eight minutes.

Carbs: 3.0 g each (6 servings recipe)

The Sweeter Side of Breakfast

Blueberry Ricotta Pancakes

Ingredients
¾ cup ricotta
3 large eggs
¼ cup unsweetened vanilla almond milk
½ teaspoon vanilla extract
½ cup golden flaxseed meal
1 teaspoon baking powder
1 cup almond flour
¼ teaspoon salt
¼ to ½ teaspoon stevia powder
¼ cup blueberries

Instructions
1. Blend the eggs, milk, ricotta, and vanilla extract with an electric mixer.
2. Combine the flaxseed meal, flour, stevia, baking powder, and salt in another dish.
3. Add the dry ingredients into the blender—slowly—to form the batter.
4. Use two to three blueberries for each pancake.
5. Add the butter to a preheated skillet. When it melts, add the batter using two tablespoons for each scoop.

Carbs: 5.9 g each (4 servings recipe)

Brownie Muffins

Ingredients
½ teaspoon salt
1 cup flaxseed meal
¼ cup cocoa powder
1 tablespoon cinnamon
½ tablespoon baking powder
1 teaspoon vanilla extract
2 tablespoons coconut oil
1 large egg
¼ cup sugar-free caramel syrup
½ cup pumpkin puree
¼ cup slivered almonds
1 teaspoon apple cider vinegar

Instructions
1. Set the oven temperature at 350°F.
2. In a deep mixing container—combine all of the ingredients. Mix well.
3. Use 6 paper liners in the muffin tin, and add ¼ cup batter to each one.
4. Sprinkle several almonds on the tops, pressing gently.
5. Bake approximately 15 minutes when the top is set.

Carbs: 3.3 g each (6 servings in the recipe)

Coconut Chia Bars

Ingredients
½ cup water
4 tablespoons chia seeds
1 tablespoon each:
- Coconut oil
- Confectioners Swerve

1 cup shredded – unsweetened- dried coconut meat
½ cup cashews
¼ teaspoon vanilla extract

Instructions
1. Set the oven temperature to 350°F.
2. Soak the seeds 15 minutes until gel-like, and mix with the coconut, oil, swerve, and vanilla extract. Lastly, add the cashews.
3. Line the mixture, using parchment paper, on a 9x9 cookie sheet. Press until it is about a ¾ inch thickness, and bake for 45 minutes. It's done when tested with a toothpick in the center and comes out clean.

Carbs: 3.5 g each (recipe is for 6 bars)

Ham and Apple Flatbread

Crust Ingredients:
¾ cup almond flour
2 cups grated mozzarella cheese (part-skim)
2 tablespoons cream cheese
1/8 teaspoon dried thyme
½ teaspoon sea salt

Topping Ingredients:
4 ounces sliced ham (low-carb)
½ small red onion
1 cup grated Mexican cheese
¼ medium apple
1/8 teaspoon dried thyme

Instructions
1. Remove the core and seeds from the apple. You can leave it unpeeled but will need to use a vegetable peeler to make thin slices.
2. Preheat the oven to 425°F.
3. Cut two pieces of parchment paper to fit into a 12-inch pizza pan (approximately two inches larger than the pan).
4. Use the high heat setting. Place a double boiler (water in the bottom pan), and bring the water to boiling. Place the heat setting on low.
5. Add the cream cheese, mozzarella cheese, salt, thyme, and almond flour to the top of the double boiler—stirring constantly.
6. When the cheese mixture resembles dough, place it on one of the pieces of parchment—and knead the dough until totally mixed.
7. Roll the dough into a ball—placing it at the center of the paper—place the second piece of paper over the top, and roll with a rolling pin (or a large glass).
8. Place the dough onto the pizza pan (leaving the paper connected).

9. Poke several holes in the dough and put into the preheated oven for approximately six to eight minutes.
10. When browned, remove it and lower the setting of the oven to 350°F.
11. Arrange the cheese, apple slices, onion slices, and ham pieces. Top off with the remainder (3/4 cup) of cheese. Flavor with the ground pepper, salt, and thyme.
12. Place in the oven and bake until the cheese melted and the crust is to the desired brown. Slide it off of the parchment paper and cool two or three minutes before cutting.

Tip: If you do not own a double boiler, you can substitute with a mixing dish over a pot of boiling water as a standby.

Carbs: 5.0 g each (8 slices)

Chapter 2: Beef Choices

Korean BBQ Keto Bowl

Ingredients
4 tablespoons Coconut Aminos
2 garlic cloves (chopped fine)
4 tablespoons Sriracha Sauce
1 teaspoon powdered ginger
2 tablespoons coconut oil
1 pound - thinly sliced - skirt steak
2 cups riced cauliflower

Instructions
1. Combine the garlic, ginger, Coconut Aminos, and Sriracha for the marinade sauce.
2. Put the steak into a zipper bag with the marinade and shake to evenly coat the pieces. Refrigerate overnight or a minimum of one hour.
3. Before cooking time (approximately 30 minutes), remove the steak from the fridge.
4. Use a non-stick pan to melt the coconut oil. Add the cauliflower and saute on the high setting for ten minutes. Stir frequently until it is browned slightly and tender.
5. Use a cast iron grill pan (10x10) on high heat to grill the meat. Grill one slice at a time for two minutes on each side, or until it is done to your satisfaction.
6. Add the steak to a serving dish with the cauliflower rice as a base.

Carbs: 3.3 g each (recipe serves 6)

Mississippi Roast – Slow Cooker

Ingredients
3.8 pounds beef chuck roast
1 (16 ounces) jar deli-sliced Greek Peperoncini
1 tablespoon each:
- Dried dill
- Garlic powder
- Onion powder
- Dried chives
- Dried parsley

¼ teaspoon black pepper
½ teaspoon salt
2 tablespoons Better than Bouillon
1 stick (1/2 cup) butter

Instructions
1. Arrange the roast in the slow cooker.
2. Drain and reserve the brine from the pepperoncini's, pouring one cup into the slow cooker, and discarding the rest.
3. Add the chives, onion powder, dried dill, garlic powder, black pepper and salt to the cooker.
4. A little at a time, add the bouillon paste. Place the butter on top of the roast and cook for 8 to 10 hours.
5. Save the juices for a later use and shred the meat.

Carbs: 3.13 g each (8 servings included)

Steak with Mushroom Port Sauce

Ingredients
2 pounds – rib-eye steak
10 ounces mushrooms
2 ounces heavy cream
1 tablespoon butter
4 ounces port wine
Pepper and salt

Instructions
1. Preheat the oven to 450°F. Flavor the rib-eye steak with pepper and salt.
2. Add the butter to a cast iron skillet on high. Cook the meat for two minutes per side. Add it to a baking pan in the oven. Cover with foil.
3. For medium rare the internal temperature will be 135°F or a total of 12 minutes, flipping ½ through the cooking cycle.
4. Pour the wine into the pan to deglaze. Add the cream and mushrooms and cook until thickened.

Carbs: 6.0 g each serving (two serving recipe)

Steak-Lovers Slow-Cooked Chili

Ingredients for Chili:
1 cup beef or chicken stock
½ cup sliced leeks
2 ½ pounds (1-inch cubes) steak
2 cups whole tomatoes (canned with juices)
1 tablespoon chili powder
½ teaspoon cumin
1/8 teaspoon ground black pepper
½ teaspoon salt
¼ teaspoon ground cayenne pepper

Optional Toppings:
1 teaspoon fresh chopped cilantro
2 tablespoons sour cream
¼ cup shredded cheddar cheese
½ avocado (cubed or sliced)

Instructions
1. Put all of the items except the topping ingredients into the slow cooker.
2. Set the cooker to high and cook for about six hours.

12 Servings per recipe
Carbs without toppings: 3.3 g per serving
Carbs with toppings: 13.49 g per serving

Ground Beef Recipes

Ground Beef Stir Fry

Ingredients
10 ½ ounces ground beef
5 medium brown mushrooms
½ cup broccoli
2 leaves kale
½ medium onion
1 tablespoon coconut oil
½ of a medium red pepper
1 tablespoon cayenne pepper
1 tablespoon Chinese Five Spices (McCormick)

Instructions
1. Prepare the veggies—slice the mushrooms and—chop the broccoli.
2. Preheat a skillet using med-high heat, place the oil and onions and cook for one minute. Combine the remainder of the vegetables and cook an additional two minutes—stir frequently.
3. Blend the spices and beef—decrease the heat to medium—and continue cooking for approximately two more minutes.
4. Cover the pan and cook for five or ten more minutes until the beef is done.
5. Serve immediately.

Carbs: 7.0 g each (recipe is for 3 servings)

Nachos or Tacos

Ingredients
17.6 ounces ground beef
1 medium white onion (3.0 ounces)
4 tacos
1 teaspoon chili powder
2 garlic cloves
½ teaspoon ground cumin
2 teaspoons extra-virgin coconut oil or ghee
1 tablespoon unsweetened tomato puree
1 cup water (8 ounces)
½ teaspoon salt—more or less
Cayenne pepper or freshly ground black pepper

Topping Ingredients:
1 small head of lettuce (approximately 3.5 ounces)
1 cup or 5.3 ounces cherry tomatoes
1 medium avocado (7.1 ounces)

Optional Toppings:
4 tablespoons sour cream
1 cup grated cheese
Veggies including cabbage, cucumbers, or peppers

Instructions
1. Using med-high, melt a small amount of butter/ghee in a pan, and add the onion. Cook until brown and mix in the beef. Continue cooking until the beef is done.
2. Add the cumin and chili powder. (You can substitute with 1 ½ teaspoon of paprika.)
3. Pour in the water and add the tomato puree. Add pepper, and salt if desired for additional flavoring.
4. Continue cooking until the meat is done and approximately ¼ of the sauce is reduced. Set aside and prepare the veggie topping.
5. Fill the shells with the meat mixture and garnish with the tomatoes, lettuce, and avocado.

Carbs: 6.6 g each (4 Servings)

Spaghetti Squash Lasagna

Ingredients
3 pounds ground beef
30 slices Mozzarella cheese
32 ounces whole milk Ricotta cheese
1 (40 ounces) jar marinara sauce
2 large – cooked – spaghetti squash (about 2 ¾ pounds)

Instructions
1. Preheat the oven temperature to 375°F.
2. Slice the squash in half. Place the halves in a cooking dish. Cover the meat portion of the squash with water, and bake for 45 minutes.
3. Brown the beef in a pan, drain and add the marinara sauce. Set aside after it's warm.
4. Scrape the meat from the squash (the spaghetti) and combine in a large baking dish as the first ingredient. Add a layer of meat sauce, Mozzarella, Ricotta, and continue until all ingredients are added.
5. Bake for 35 minutes until the cheese is browned.

Carbs: 15.0 g each (recipe is 12 servings)

Hamburger Stroganoff

Ingredients
8 ounces sliced mushrooms
1 pound ground beef
2 minced cloves of garlic
2 tablespoons butter
1 teaspoon lemon juice
1 ¼ cups sour cream
1/3 cup water or dry white wine
¼ teaspoon paprika
1 teaspoon dried parsley/*Substitute*: 1 tablespoon chopped fresh parsley

Instructions
1. Use a frying pan to sauté the onions and garlic using one tablespoon of butter. Mix in the beef, and add some pepper and salt if desired. Cook until done and set to the side.
2. Use the remainder of the butter, the mushrooms, and the wine/water—add them to the pan. Cook until half of the liquid is reduced and the mushrooms are soft. Take them off the burner—add the paprika and sour cream.
3. On low heat stir in the meat and lemon juice. Use additional spices for flavoring if desired.

Carbs: 6.1 g (recipe for 4 servings

Sweet and Sour Meatballs

Ingredients for the Meatballs
1 pound ground beef (30 mini balls)
1 large egg
½ teaspoon onion powder
¼ cup Parmesan cheese

Ingredients for the Sauce
¼ cup apple cider vinegar
1 ½ cups water
¼ cup sugar-free ketchup
3 tablespoons soy sauce

Instructions
1. Combine all of the meatball ingredients. Use a tablespoon to shape the meatballs.
2. Use medium heat in a saucepan and cook the meatballs until browned (slightly pink centers). Set aside.
3. Pour the rest of the ingredients. Gently whisk the ingredients.
4. Lower the heat and simmer to thicken, adding the meatballs. Cook about ten more minutes on the low setting.

Carbs: 5.35 g each (5 servings)

Chapter 3: Chicken - Duck - and Turkey Choices

Chicken—Broccoli—Zucchini Boats

Ingredients
6 ounces shredded chicken
2 tablespoons butter
2 hollowed-out zucchini (10 ounces)
3 ounces shredded cheddar cheese
1 stalk of green onion
1 cup broccoli
2 tablespoons sour cream

Instructions
1. Program the oven temperature to 400°F.
2. Slice the zucchini lengthwise and scoop most of the insides until you have a shell of approximately ½ to 1 cm. thick.
3. Melt one tablespoon of the butter into each boat, flavor with a dash of pepper and salt if you wish, and bake them for around twenty minutes.
4. Shred the chicken, cut the broccoli florets into small pieces, and measure out six ounces of cheese. Mix with the sour cream.
5. Remove the zucchini shells when done and add the mixture.
6. Sprinkle each of them with the remainder of the cheese.
7. Bake for another ten or fifteen minutes until the cheese is browned and melted.
8. Use a bit of mayo, sour cream, or chopped onion as a garnish.

Carbs: 8g each (recipe provides 2 servings)

Chicken Smothered in Creamy Onion Sauce

Ingredients
1 whole green/spring onion
2 tablespoons or 1-ounce butter
4 chicken breast halves – skinless - boneless (approx. 6 ounces)
8 ounces sour cream
½ teaspoon sea salt

Instructions
1. Use the med-high setting to melt the butter in a large pan. Lower the setting to med-low—place the chicken with the butter—cover and cook about ten additional minutes.
2. Chop the onion using the white and green sections.
3. Flip the breasts—cover and simmer—another eight or nine minutes (or until completely done).
4. Combine the onion and continue cooking one or two minutes.
5. Take it off of the burner, and blend in the sour cream and salt.
6. Let the meal rest for five minutes. Blend well and serve.

Carbs: 3.3 g each (recipe is 4 servings)

Chicken Stuffed Avocado—Cajun Style

Ingredients
1 ½ cups cooked chicken (7.4 ounces)
2 medium or 1 large avocados (10.6 ounces)
2 tablespoons cream cheese/sour cream
2 tablespoons lemon juice (fresh)
¼ cup mayonnaise
½ teaspoon each: onion powder & garlic powder
¼ teaspoon each: salt (more or less) and cayenne pepper
1 teaspoon each: paprika and dried thyme

Instructions
1. Shred the chicken into small pieces.
2. Combine all of the ingredients—saving the salt and lemon juice until last.
3. Leave one-half to one-inch of the avocado flesh—scoop the middle. Remove the seeds.
4. Cut the center/scooped pieces of avocado into small pieces and fill the halves with the mixture of chicken.

Carbs: 5.4 g each (recipe is 2 servings)

Creamy Chicken Casserole

Ingredients
2 pounds chicken thighs
7 ounces shredded cheese
2/3 pound cauliflower florets
1 leek
4 ounces cherry tomatoes
1 ¼ cups sour cream or heavy whipping cream
2 tablespoons green pesto
3 tablespoons butter
 ½ lemon (the juice)
Pepper and salt

Instructions
1. Program the oven to 400°F.
2. Combine the pesto, cream, and lemon juice. Add pepper and salt for flavoring.
3. Fry the chicken in the butter until browned and transfer to a baking dish. Pour in the mixture.
4. Chop the tomatoes and leek and add to the top of the chicken along with the cauliflower. Sprinkle the cheese on the top and bake until the chicken is done (a minimum of 30 minutes).

Carbs: 7.0 g each (4 serving recipe)

Roasted Chicken

Ingredients
1 whole chicken
2 rosemary sprigs
2 garlic cloves
1 teaspoon Herbes de Provence spice
1 tablespoon coarse sea salt

Instructions
1. Program the oven to 350°F. Rinse and arrange the *room temperature* chicken in a Pyrex dish – breast side up.
2. Add the rosemary and cloves in the chicken cavity. Drizzle with the spice and salt. Bake 1 ½ hours until browned.

Carbs: 0.0 each (8 servings recipe)

Turducken

Ingredients
1 chicken
1 duck
1 turkey
6 sausage links
2 egg yolks
¾ cup almond flour
1 diced green pepper
1 diced onion
4 diced celery stalks
To taste: Poultry seasoning

Instructions for the Meat Stuffing
1. Cook the sausage and add the chopped vegetables.
2. Combine the flour, veggies, and sausage in a large mixing dish and add the yolks, mixing thoroughly.

Instructions for the Turducken
1. Debone the duck and chicken. Also, debone the chicken but leave the wings and legs intact.
2. Season the entire surfaces of all meats.
3. Arrange the turkey in a baking dish and layer it with the stuffing mixture.
4. Place the duck down with legs in the opposite direction of the turkey and add stuffing.
5. Do the same with the chicken with the legs in the same direction of the turkey and layer with more stuffing.
6. Pull the two sides of chicken together and use skewers to close. Do the same with the duck and turkey.
7. Tie the turkey with some kitchen twine
8. Cook at 500°F for 15 minutes. Reduce the heat and cook for 300°F for 6 hours (internal temperature will be 165°F).
9. Slice the Turducken into slices, so each has a serving of stuffing

Carbs: 3.0 g each (24 servings in the recipe)

Roasted Duck

Ingredients
1 Duck

Instructions

1. Preheat the oven to 300F.
2. Discard any excess fat from the thawed duck. Remove any extras in the carcass and tie the legs together with some kitchen twine.
3. Arrange in a baking pan and cook for three hours. Poke the skin occasionally with a sharp knife.
4. Slice into quarters and serve.

Carbs: 0.0 g each (4 servings in the recipe)

Skillet Style Sausage and Cabbage Melt

Ingredients
4 spicy Italian chicken sausages
2 tablespoons coconut oil
½ cup diced onion
1 ½ cups purple cabbage
1 ½ cups green cabbage
2 tablespoons chopped fresh cilantro
2 (1-ounce) slices Colby Jack cheese

Instructions
1. Begin by removing the sausage casings and roughly chop them.
2. Shred the cabbage and chop the onions.
3. Add the coconut oil, cabbage, and onion in a large skillet using the med-high setting for approximately eight minutes (the veggies should be tender).
4. Blend the cheese and cover. Turn the heat off and let it rest five minutes as the cheese melts.
5. When it is time to serve—stir gently—and add the cilantro.

Carbs: 3.52 g each (4 servings)

Chapter 4: Pork Choices

Keto Rack of Ribs

Ingredients
2 racks of ribs (6.72 pounds)
2 tablespoons paprika
½ teaspoon stevia (more or less)
1 tablespoon each:
- Salt
- Garlic powder

½ tablespoon each:
- Ground ginger
- Pepper
- Onion powder

¼ tablespoon cayenne pepper
2 ounces Dijon mustard

Instructions
1. Set the oven temperature to 225°F.
2. Cut away any membrane on the back of the ribs.
3. Combine all of the spices and rub it into the meat. Add them to a foil-lined baking sheet and bake uncovered for 60 minutes.
4. Cook for 3 ½ more hours by adding an aluminum foil tent. Turn after two hours. When done, the internal temperature should be 180°F.
5. Discard the foil and broil on high for five minutes for a brown crust.
6. Cover for ten minutes before serving.

Carbs: 4.0 g (one serving 4 ribs)

Spaghetti Squash Meatballs

Ingredients
2 spaghetti squash
32 ounces ground pork
1 small onion
1 egg
1 tablespoon ground flax seed
8 ounces Mozzarella cheese
½ teaspoon each:
- Onion powder
- Garlic powder
- Black pepper
- Salt
- Worcestershire sauce
- Hot sauce

2 ounces grated parmesan cheese
3 cups tomato basil sauce

Instructions
1. Program the oven to 375°F.
2. Prepare the squash (cut in half and remove seeds).
3. Place face down in a Pyrex dish with 2 cups of water, and bake 45 minutes.
4. Combine the egg, pork, flax seed, spices, and parmesan cheese.
5. Shape the meat into 2 ounce balls, and cut the mozzarella into 18 equal pieces.
6. Add a piece to the center of each of the meatballs.
7. Arrange them on a baking sheet for 25 minutes.
8. Shred the squash when done and mix in the sauce and meatballs.

Carbs: 17.0 g each (6 servings in the recipe)
    One serving = 3 meatballs, 1 cup spaghetti, and ½ cup sauce

Squash and Sausage Casserole

Ingredients
1 pound browned sausage
2 large eggs
1 medium zucchini (sliced & cooked)
2 medium summer squash (sliced & cooked)
1 teaspoon salt
½ teaspoon onion powder or ¼ cup dried minced onion
1 cup mayonnaise
1 package sugar substitute (or stevia)
¼ teaspoon pepper
1 ½ cups shredded cheddar cheese (divided)
¼ melted butter

Instructions
1. Preheat the oven to 350°F.
2. Combine each of the ingredients except for ½ cup of shredded cheese.
3. Place the ingredients into a lightly greased 9 x 13 x 2 baking dish.
4. Sprinkle the remainder of cheese on the casserole. Bake until lightly browned for approximately 30 minutes.

Carbs: 2.0 g (1 serving = 124 g or 4.4 ounces approximately)
12 servings in the recipe

Sunflower Pork & Butter Kabobs

Ingredients for the Marinade
2 teaspoons hot sauce
3 tablespoons sunflower butter
½ teaspoon crushed red pepper
1 tablespoon each:
- Soy sauce
- Minced garlic
- Water

1 pound pork kabob squares
1 medium green pepper

Instructions
1. Cube the kabobs and green pepper into squares.
2. Use a food processor for the marinade ingredients, and process until smooth.
3. Combine the squares of pork with the marinade overnight, or a minimum of one hour in a non-metal dish.
4. Thread the pork and peppers onto metal skewers and broil five minutes per side until the internal temperature is 145°F.

Carbs: 5.0 g per kabob (4 serving recipe)

Tenderloin Stuffed Keto Style

Ingredients
2 pounds pork tenderloin or venison
½ cup feta cheese
½ cup gorgonzola cheese
1 teaspoon chopped onion
2 tablespoons crushed almonds
2 garlic cloves, minced
½ teaspoon each: fresh ground black pepper and sea salt

Instructions
1. Preheat the grill.
2. Form a pocket in the tenderloin.
3. Mix the cheeses, almonds, garlic, and onions. Stuff and seal the pocket using a skewer.
4. Grill until you are satisfied with its doneness.

Carbs: 2.8 g each (4 servings in recipe)

Thai Pork Salad with Kelp Noodles

Ingredients
1 pound ground pork (20%fat)
1 tablespoon lard/virgin coconut oil/tallow
1.2 ounces mixed minced herbs (cilantro, mint, Thai basil)
2-inch piece (0.4 ounces) piece of fresh minced ginger
3 minced garlic cloves (0.5 ounces)
2 small thinly sliced shallots (1.1 ounces)
4 thinly sliced onions (1.1 ounces)
1 tablespoon fish sauce
3 tablespoons – juice of 1 lime
1 teaspoon - zest of 1 lime
1 tablespoon coconut aminos
1 teaspoon red pepper flakes
½ teaspoon white pepper
1 (12 ounces) bag kelp noodles
For serving: Lettuce cups (3 ounces)

Instructions
1. Use a skillet on high heat to warm the fat. Toss in the shallot and pork to cook for six to eight minutes – breaking it apart with a wooden spoon until browned.
2. Blend the minced ginger, garlic, green onions, and ½ of the herbs in a mixing container.
3. Add the coconut aminos, fish sauce, zest and juice of the lime, white pepper, and pepper flakes in a separate dish.
4. Combine the herb mixture to the skillet and cook one minute and add the sauce.
5. Turn the heat off and stir in the remainder of herbs. Add a pinch of salt if desired.
6. Prepare the salad with the lettuce cups, and kelp noodles for a special dish.

Carbs: 9.3 g each serving (recipe for 2 servings)

Chapter 5: Seafood Recipes

Baked Salmon

Ingredients
2 (6 ounces) salmon fillets
6 tablespoons light olive oil
1 teaspoon each:
- Salt
- Ground black pepper
- Dried basil

1 tablespoon each:
- Chopped fresh parsley
- Lemon juice

Instructions
1. Preheat the oven to 375°F.
2. Prepare the marinade (with all of the ingredients) and add the fillets in a medium glass dish. Let it rest for one hour, rotating occasionally.
3. Arrange the fillets in aluminum foil, cover with the marinade, and close.
4. Bake 35 to 45 minutes.

Carbs: 2.0 g each serving (2 servings)

Coconut Shrimp

Ingredients
1 pound shrimp
2 large egg whites
2 tablespoons coconut flour
1 cup unsweetened coconut flakes

Sweet Chili Dipping Sauce
1 ½ tablespoons wine vinegar
½ cup sugar-free apricot preserves
1 medium diced red chili
1 tablespoon lime juice
¼ teaspoon red pepper flakes

Instructions
1. Preheat the oven to 400°F.
2. Peel and devein the shrimp.
3. Beat the eggs to form soft peaks. Arrange the coconut flakes and flour into individual bowls.
4. Dip the shrimp in the flour, egg mixture, and coconut flakes.
5. Place them on a lightly greased baking sheet of silpat for fifteen minutes. Flip them and broil another three to five minutes on each side.
6. Combine the dipping sauce and stir well.

Carbs: 6.5 g each (3 servings shrimp and 2 ½ tablespoons sauce)
The recipe is for 5 servings.

Rockfish with Creamy Ginger Avocado Dressing

Ingredients
1 pound rockfish or cod (4 fillets)
2 egg whites
½ teaspoon sea salt
1/3 cup coconut flour
3 tablespoons coconut oil

Dressing Ingredients
½ cup coconut cream
½ tablespoon chopped fresh cilantro
½ teaspoon grated fresh ginger
1/3 fresh serrano pepper
1 teaspoon each:
- Sea salt
- Fresh lemon juice

1 medium avocado

Instructions
1. Deseed the pepper for a less spicy dish.
2. Whisk the eggs and salt. Sieve the coconut flour to remove chunks. Dip the fish into the eggs and flour.
3. Cook in the coconut oil over a high setting for two minutes, flip, and add more oil if necessary.
4. Reduce the heat for another three minutes and serve.
5. *For the Dressing*: Use a food processor on high and blend the ingredients until creamy smooth. Add about two tablespoons of dressing over the top of each fish.

Carbs: 2.0 g (4 serving recipe)

Sardine Fritters

Ingredients
½ cup psyllium
1 can (6 ounces) sardines – oil drained
4 beaten eggs
½ teaspoon salt
2 cups cilantro
½ cup coconut flour (dredging)
4 tablespoons coconut oil (frying)

Instructions
1. Mash the sardines to bits and add the psyllium, salt, and eggs. Let it set for about five minutes.
2. Wash and chop the cilantro and add it to the bowl.
3. Form the dough into 12 patties, approximately ¾-inches thick and 2-inches in diameter. Dredge them in the flour.
4. Heat one tablespoon of oil in a non-stick or ceramic skillet. Fry only three at a time, three to four minutes per side.
5. Use a spatula to flatten the fritters. Drain on a towel and serve cold or hot.

Carbs: 1.8 g (3 patties are one serving)
   Note: The recipe is for 12 patties.

Tuna Avocado Melt

Ingredients
1 (10 ounces) can drained tuna
1 medium cubed avocado
¼ cup mayonnaise (see recipe in sauces)
1/3 cup almond flour
¼ teaspoon onion powder
¼ cup parmesan cheese
½ teaspoon garlic powder
1/2 cup coconut oil (for frying)

Instructions
1. In a container, blend all of the ingredients except the coconut oil and avocado.
2. Fold the cubed avocado into the tuna.
3. Make balls and coat each one with the almond flour.
4. Use the medium heat setting and place the oil in a skillet—mix the tuna—and continue cooking until brown.

Carbs: 0.8 g each (12 melt bites per recipe)

Chapter 6: Salads–Sides–Sauces–Soups–and Snacks

Salads

Asparagus and Radish Salad

Ingredients
1 ½ pounds asparagus spears
1 teaspoon parsley
10 radishes
4 ounces sour cream
1 tablespoon each:
- Olive oil
- Mayonnaise
- Lemon juice
- Dill

1 teaspoon white wine vinegar
Pepper

Instructions
1. Prepare the asparagus spears by washing and removing the woody end.
2. Add them to boiling – salted water for two or three minutes (until bright green). Stop the cooking process by dropping them in a pot of ice water. Cut them into one-inch sections.
3. Prepare the radishes by removing the ends and use a mandolin for thin slices.
4. Blend the remainder of the ingredients in a food processor to make the dressing.

Carbs: 9.0 grams (4 servings in the recipe)

Avocado and Bacon Salad

Ingredients
2 small heads lettuce (7 ounces)
2 large avocados (14 ounces)
1 medium spring onion (1/2 ounce)
2 cups fresh spinach (2 ounces)
4 large bacon slices (4 ounces)

Vinaigrette Dressing
3 tablespoons extra virgin olive oil
1 tablespoon apple cider vinegar
1 teaspoon Dijon mustard
Pepper and a pinch of salt (Pink Himalayan)
Option: Dash of Tabasco

Instructions
1. Combine the ingredients. Add the vinaigrette.
2. *Note*: Keep in mind that the ounces are provided as an estimate for your salad intake.

Carbs: 6.7 each (two servings in the recipe - with dressing)

Bistro Steak Salad with Horseradish Dressing

Ingredients
1 (12 ounces) rib-eye steak
¼ teaspoon each:
  - Pepper
  - Salt
1 (7 ounces) bag romaine salad greens
1 (2.1 ounces) small thinly sliced red onion
4 slices uncured bacon
4.2 ounces cherry tomatoes
½ cup (2 ounces) sliced radishes

For the Dressing
2 tablespoons prepared horseradish
¼ cup mayonnaise (see sauces)
Pepper and salt

Instructions
1. Line a baking sheet with parchment paper and program the oven to 350°F.
2. Arrange the bacon (single-layered) in the pan and bake for 15 minutes. Drain and break into bits.
3. Pat the steak with some towels and flavor with the pepper and salt.
4. Grill four minutes and flip, cooking another 12 to 15 minutes (Medium is 12 minutes with an internal temperature of 155°F.) Wait five minutes and slice against the grain into small slices.
5. Prepare the dressing and enjoy.

Carbs: 6.2 g per serving (recipe for 2 servings)

Bok-Choy Salad – Oven-Baked

Tofu Ingredients
15 ounces extra firm tofu
2 teaspoons minced garlic
Juice from ½ a lemon
1 tablespoon each:
- sesame oil
- water
- soy sauce
- rice wine vinegar

Bok Choy Salad Ingredients
2 tablespoons soy sauce
1 stalk green onion
2 tablespoons chopped cilantro
9 ounces bok choy
3 tablespoons coconut oil
1 tablespoon Sambal Olek
Juice of ½ of a lime
1 tablespoon peanut butter
7 drops liquid Stevia

Instructions
1. You will need to press the tofu in towels for approximately five to six hours to dry.
2. Combine each of the marinade ingredients.
3. When dry, chop the tofu into squares and put in a plastic container/bag with the marinade sauce. Leave it to rest for a minimum of thirty minutes—preferably overnight.
4. Preheat the oven to 350°F. Bake for 30 to 35 minutes on a parchment paper lined baking dish or a silpat (non-stick baking sheet with a blend of fiberglass mesh and silicone).
5. Meanwhile, mix the dressing ingredients (except for the bok choy) in a mixing dish. Add the onion and cilantro.
6. Chop the bok choy as you would cabbage, into small slices.
7. Remove the tofu—combine, and enjoy.

Note: Bok choy is a Chinese vegetable.
Carbs: 7.3 g each (recipe is 3 servings)

Mixed Green Spring Salad

Ingredients
2 ounces mixed greens
3 tablespoons roasted pine nuts
2 tablespoons Vinaigrette (above)
2 tablespoons shaved Parmesan cheese
2 bacon slices
Pepper and salt

Instructions
1. Prepare the bacon and crumble it in the salad along with the remainder of the ingredients.
2. Sprinkle with the Vinaigrette dressing and serve.

Carbs: 4.3 g per serving (recipe is one serving with dressing)

Zucchini and Walnut Salad

Ingredients
1 tablespoon olive oil
2 zucchinis
3 ½ ounces arugula lettuce
1 head romaine lettuce
5 1/3 tablespoons finely chopped scallions or chives
¾ cup chopped pecans or walnuts
Pepper and salt

Ingredients for the Dressing
¾ cup mayonnaise (recipe under sauces)
2 tablespoons olive oil
1 clove of garlic
¼ teaspoon chili powder
½ teaspoon salt

Instructions
1. Whisk the dressing ingredients in a small container.
2. Slice the zucchini lengthwise and remove the seeds. Cut the halves crosswise, making ½-inch sections.
3. Using a skillet (medium heat), add the oil. Toss in the zucchini, pepper, and salt, sautéing until browned, yet firm.
4. Trim the salad and add the arugula, romaine, and chives in a bowl, and add to the zucchini mixture.
5. Roast the nuts a minute or so, in the same pan as the zucchini, and season with pepper and salt. Scoop the nuts onto the salad and sprinkle with the dressing.

Carbs: 2.0 g each (4 servings in the recipe)

Veggies and Sides

Deep-Fat Fried and Spicy Brussels Sprouts

Ingredients
1 ½ pounds Brussels sprouts
2 ounces mayonnaise (recipe listed with sauces)
½ ounce Sriracha sauce
1 teaspoon lime juice

Instructions
1. Prepare, wash, and quarter the Brussels sprouts.
2. Deep fry the sprouts in batches for six minutes (do not overload).
3. Combine with the remainder of ingredients and enjoy.

Carbs: 16.0 carbs each (4 servings in recipe)

Cauliflower Hash Browns

Ingredients
1 pound cauliflower
½ yellow onion - grated
3 eggs
2 pinches – pepper
1 teaspoon salt
For frying: 4 ounces butter

Instructions
1. Discard the leaves and coarsely shred/crumble 16 ounces of cauliflower.
2. Combine the mix with the remainder of the ingredients. Let it rest five to ten minutes.
3. Heat the butter in a skillet. Cook about 3 to 4 at a time.
4. Scoop the mixture into the frying pan, and carefully flatten each one into a 3 to 4-inch patty.
5. Fry each side for four to five minutes. (Don't flip too frequently because they will crumble.)

Carbs: 5.0 g each (4 servings in the recipe)

Cauliflower Rice

Ingredients
1 2/3 pounds cauliflower
½ teaspoon salt
3 ¼ ounces coconut oil/butter
Optional: ½ teaspoon turmeric

Instructions
1. Grate the head of cauliflower (the rice).
2. Melt the oil/butter in a skillet over medium heat for about five to ten minutes until the rice is softened. Toss in the salt and turmeric.

Microwave Instructions
1. Place the rice in a glass dish and cover with some plastic wrap for five to six minutes.
2. Add the butter/oil to melt.

Carbs: 5.0 g each (4 servings in recipe)

Keto Cole Slaw

Ingredients
½ of a lemon (the juice)
¼ green cabbage
1 teaspoon salt
6 ¾ tablespoons mayonnaise (see recipe under sauces)
1 tablespoon Dijon mustard
Pinch of pepper
Optional: Pinch fennel seeds

Instructions
1. Core and shred the cabbage with a cheese slicer or food processor in a container.
2. Add the lemon juice and salt. Stir and set aside for ten minutes (remove excess liquid).
3. Combine the cabbage, mayonnaise, and mustard (if using).

Carbs: 2.0 g each (4 servings in the recipe)

Southern Fried Cabbage

Ingredients
1 ½ pounds white cabbage
8 slices raw bacon
1 large chopped onion
½ teaspoon black pepper
1 teaspoon sea salt or Himalayan salt
Optional: 5 drops liquid stevia

Instructions
1. Remove the core and shred the cabbage. Cook the bacon over medium-high heat, and chop. Save the bacon fat.
2. Lower the heat and fry the onion five to ten minutes until caramelized.
3. Add the cabbage and increase the heat to the medium setting for about 15 minutes. Stir about every five minutes.
4. Add the pepper and salt along with the stevia if you prefer a sweeter cabbage.

Carbs: 4.3 g each (six servings in recipe)

Spaghetti Squash

Ingredients
1 squash

Instructions
1. Preheat the oven to 375°F.
2. Rinse the squash and slice it lengthwise. Scoop out and discard the seeds.
3. Arrange the squash face down in a baking dish. Pour about ½ to 1-inch of water to the dish. Bake 30 to 45 minutes.
4. The squash is done when the spaghetti is easily removed.
5. Sauté the squash in some oil and garlic or top it with some sauce.

Carbs: 10.g (1 cup serving)

Stuffed Green Peppers – Keto Style

Ingredients
2 sausage links
2 green peppers
1 small onion
2 ounces cream cheese
1 ½ ounces Parmesan cheese
2 quail eggs
1 chicken egg

Instructions
1. Program the oven to 400°F.
2. Cut away the sausage skin and cook it until crumbly. Drain the grease on towels.
3. Remove the pepper tops and discard the seeds.
4. Chop the peppers and onions and cook in a skillet. Combine the mix with the cream cheese, chicken egg, and sausage.
5. Stuff the peppers, and top it off with a quail egg.
6. Bake for 20 minutes.

Carbs: 14 carbs each (2 servings provided)

Sauces

Low-Carb Mayonnaise

Ingredients
1 egg yolk
1 tablespoon Dijon mustard
1 to 2 teaspoons white vinegar/lemon juice
1 cup light olive oil

Instructions
1. In advance, allow the mustard and egg to become room temperature. Use a mixer/stick blender to combine the mustard and egg.
2. Slowly, add the oil until the mixture thickens.
3. Add the lemon juice/vinegar. Mix well and add a pinch of salt and pepper if desired for additional flavoring.

Note: Use white wine vinegar or lemon juice for seafood. For roast beef or cold cuts use the red wine vinegar – not balsamic.

Carbs: 0.0 g (recipe for 4 servings)

Soups

Beef Bone Broth – Slow Cooker

Ingredients
3 to 4 pounds mixed bones (neck bones, oxtail, short ribs, etc.)
2 medium onions
3 celery stalks
2 medium carrots
1 bay leaf
1 tablespoon olive oil
2 tablespoons apple cider vinegar

Instructions
1. Coarsely chop the onions, celery, and carrots.
2. Heat the oven temperature to 400°F.
3. In a roasting pan, layer the bones and drizzle with the oil. Bake 30 minutes, flip, and roast another 30 minutes.
4. Arrange all of the ingredients in the slow cooker or soup pot. Cover the mixture with water, and simmer for approximately 12 hours.

Yields: 2 quarts
Carbs: 1.0 g each (Serving size of 16 ounces)

Cauliflower Soup with Crumbled Pancetta

Ingredients
1 pound cauliflower
3 ¾ cups vegetable or chicken stock
7 ¾ ounces cream cheese
4 ounces butter
1 tablespoon Dijon mustard
Pepper and salt
7 ¾ ounces – diced - bacon or pancetta
1 teaspoon smoked chili or paprika powder
3 ½ ounces pecan nuts
For frying: 1 tablespoon butter (in addition)

Instructions
1. Trim and prepare the cauliflower into small florets, reserving a small handful.
2. Use a skillet to sauté the pancetta and cauliflower in the butter. Towards the end, add the paprika and nuts. Save the fat.
3. Prepare the florets until softened. Add the cream cheese, butter, and mustard. Use a mixer to reach the desired consistency and add a pinch of pepper and salt if desired.
4. Crumble some pancetta or floret crumbles to garnish.

Carbs: 5.0 g each (recipe for 4 servings)

Chicken and Chili – Crock Pot

Ingredients
1 green pepper
2 tablespoons unsalted butter
1 onion (8.8 ounces)
8 boneless chicken thighs
8 bacon slices
1 tablespoon thyme
1 teaspoon each pepper and salt
1 tablespoon each:
- Minced garlic
- Coconut flour

3 tablespoons lemon juice
¼ cup unsweetened coconut milk
1 cup chicken stock
3 tablespoons tomato paste

Instructions
1. Add the butter to the slow cooker and add the thinly sliced peppers and onions.
2. Arrange the thighs, and add the diced slices of bacon. Toss in the pepper, salt, coconut flour, thyme, and garlic.
3. Empty the milk, chicken stock, lemon juice, and tomato paste.
4. Set the cooker for six hours.
5. Stir to complete break apart the chicken before serving.

Note: You can mix the ingredients before adding them to the pot if you wish.
Carbs: 7.0 g each serving (8 servings)

Chorizo and Chicken Soup - Crock Pot

Ingredients
1 pound chorizo
4 pounds chicken thighs (no bones or skin)
4 cups chicken stock
1 large can stewed tomatoes
1 cup heavy cream
2 tablespoons each:
- Minced garlic
- Worcestershire sauce
- Hot sauce

Garnish: Shaved Parmesan cheese and sour cream

Instructions
1. Use a skillet to brown the chorizo.
2. Layer the raw chicken in the pot, the chorizo, and the rest of the ingredients.
3. Cook for three hours on high. Break the thighs apart, and return them to the pot, cooking on low for 30 additional minutes.
4. Garnish with the sour cream and Parmesan cheese.

Carbs: 6.0 each (8 servings in the recipe)

Snacks

Bacon Wrapped Scallops

Ingredients
12 thin bacon slices
12 scallops
Pepper and salt
1 tablespoon oil or bacon fat
12 toothpicks

Instructions
1. Use the high setting, and pour the oil/fat in a skillet.
2. Wrap each of the scallops with a slice of bacon, pierced with a toothpick.
3. Sprinkle with the pepper and salt. Cook for 2 ½ minutes on each side.

Carbs: 3.0 g for 4 scallops (recipe serves 4)

Beef and Bacon Rolls

Ingredients
4 bacon slices
16 ounces stew beef/steak
Steak seasoning

Instructions
1. Heat the oil in a deep fryer to 370°F.
2. Slice the beef into 1x1x2-inch cubes (1 ounce each).
3. Stretch and cut each slice of the bacon into four pieces.
4. Use the steak seasoning to flavor the beef.
5. Wrap the bacon around each piece of steak and place on a skewer.
6. Cook three minutes.

Carbs: 0 g (serving size 4 pieces) Recipe serves 4

Mini Eggplant Pizza – Keto

Ingredients
1 large eggplant
2 cups shredded Mozzarella cheese
4 tablespoons extra virgin olive oil
1 cup low-carb tomato sauce
To taste: Oregano, pepper, and salt
Toppings: Sausage, pepperoni, basil, onion, green pepper, etc.

Instructions
1. Program the oven to 375°F.
2. Slice the eggplant into ½-inch rounds and flavor with the oregano, pepper, and salt.
3. Drizzle with olive oil and bake for approximately 15 minutes. Remove them and flip to top with the tomato sauce, cheese, and additional toppings.
4. Add them to the oven broiler for five minutes or until the cheese is bubbly.

Carbs: 6.2 g each (4 servings – 2 pizzas per serving)
Note: Additional toppings should be precooked, and are already added in the carb counts. Be sure to count any additional items for the carbohydrate counts.

Pizza Base

Ingredients
3 eggs
2 teaspoons almond meal salt/red pepper flakes/pepper
2 tablespoons coconut flour
Toppings of your choice

Instructions
1. Set the oven to 350°F.
2. Mix the ingredients into a batter. Place some butter in a skillet, add the batter, and cover.
3. As the bubbles appear, flip it, and cook for about one to two minutes.
4. Cool the base, add your toppings, and cook for five to six minutes.

Carbs: 4.5 net carbs (1 serving recipe for the base only)

Raw Spiraled Zucchini Noodles with Tomatoes and Pesto

Ingredients for the Pesto
1 cup packed fresh basil
1 garlic clove
¼ cup fresh grated Parmesan cheese
Pepper and Salt
3 tablespoons extra virgin olive oil

Ingredients for the Zoodles
4 small or 3 medium zucchinis (21 ounces approximately)
Black pepper and kosher salt
1 cup halved grape or cherry tomatoes

Instructions
1. Pulse the pepper, salt, garlic, basil, and Parmesan cheese in a food processor. Pour the oil in slowly while pulsing.
2. Slice the zucchini into spirals and arrange them in a wok dish.
3. Toss gently with the tomatoes and pesto. Use a shake of pepper and salt if desired.

Carbs: 9.0 g each - 1 ¼ cup serving (recipe is 4 servings)

Zucchini and Goat Cheese Wraps

Instructions
6 ounces soft goat cheese
1 zucchini
1 teaspoon dill
Pepper and salt
1 teaspoon dried mint
Oil

Ingredients
1. Wash the zucchini and remove the ends. Slice it with a mandolin into
   1/8-inch slices.
2. Cover the slices with oil, pepper, and salt.
3. Grill each side for 2 ½ minutes (total of five minutes).
4. Mix the mint, dill, and cheese, and add to the slices of zucchini.
5. Roll each one up and secure it with a toothpick.

Carbs: 3.0 each (recipe for 6 wraps)

Chapter 7: Desserts

Brownie Cheesecake

The Brownie Base Ingredients
2 ounces chopped unsweetened chocolate
2 large eggs
½ cup butter
1/2 cup almond flour
1 pinch of salt
¼ cup cocoa powder
¾ cup granulated Erythritol/Swerve Sweetener
¼ cup chopped pecans/walnuts
¼ teaspoon vanilla

Cheesecake Filling Ingredients
2 large eggs
1 pound softened cream cheese
½ cup granulated sugar/Swerve sweetener
½ teaspoon vanilla extract
 ¼ cup heavy cream

Instructions
1. Butter a nine-inch springform pan, wrapping the bottom with foil.
2. Set the oven at 325°F.
3. Begin by melting the chocolate and butter in a microwave-safe dish for 30 seconds.
4. Whisk the cocoa powder, almond flour, and salt in a small dish.
5. In a separate dish, whip the vanilla, eggs, and Swerve until smooth.
6. Blend the flour mixture and chocolate/butter mixture. Blend in the nuts.
7. Spread out in the prepared dish and bake for approximately 15 to 20 minutes.
8. Let it cool for about 20 to 25 minutes.

For the Filling

1. Lower the oven setting to 300°F.
2. In a large mixing container - blend Swerve, the cream cheese, cream, eggs, and vanilla until everything is thoroughly mixed.
3. Empty the filling ingredients into the crust and place it on a large cookie sheet. Bake for about 35 to 45 minutes. The center should barely jiggle.
4. Loosen the edges with a knife. Place them in the fridge for a minimum of three hours.

Carbs: 6.71 g each (10 servings in the recipe)

No-Bake Cashew Coconut Bars

Ingredients
¼ cup maple syrup/sugar-free
1 cup almond flour
¼ cup melted butter
1 teaspoon cinnamon
½ cup cashews
A pinch of salt
1/4 cup shredded coconut

Instructions
1. Mix the flour and melted butter in a large mixing dish.
2. Add the maple syrup, cinnamon, salt, and coconut—blend well.
3. Use roasted or raw cashews. Chop them and add to the cashew-coconut bar dough. Blend well again.
4. Cover a cookie pan with parchment paper and spread the dough onto the paper in an even layer.
5. Place in the fridge for a minimum of two hours. Slice them and enjoy.

Carbs: 6.1 g each (8 servings in the recipe)

Cheesecake Lemon Mousse

Ingredients
2 lemons—or 1/4 cup lemon juice
1 cup heavy cream
8 ounces cream cheese
1/8 teaspoon salt
½ to 1 teaspoon lemon liquid Stevia

Instructions
1. In a standing mixer, combine the lemon juice and cream cheese until smooth. Add the remainder of the ingredients and whip until blended.
2. Adjust the flavor/sweetener if desired. Place into some serving dishes and sprinkle with some lemon zest.
3. Refrigerate until you are ready to enjoy.

Carbs: 1.7 g each (5 servings in the recipe)

Chocolate Silk Pie

Ingredients for the Crust:
1 teaspoon butter (grease the pan)
3 tablespoons butter/crust
1 ½ teaspoons vanilla extract
1 medium egg
1/3 cup granulated stevia/erythritol (sugar substitute)
1 ½ cups of almond flour
½ teaspoon baking powder
1/8 teaspoon salt

For the Filling:
4 tablespoons butter
16 ounces cream cheese – room temperature
½ cup cocoa powder
1/2 cup (+) 2 teaspoons granulated stevia
4 tablespoons sour cream
1 tablespoon vanilla extract
1 cup whipping cream
1 additional teaspoon vanilla extract for whipped cream

Instructions
1. Program the oven to 375°F. Use one teaspoon of butter to grease a nine-inch pan.
2. Combine the salt, 1/3 cup stevia, flour, and baking powder in a container.
3. Whisk the dry components and add the butter using a whisk, fork, or pastry blender to make coarse crumbs.
4. Add the vanilla extract and egg until balls are formed from the dough.
5. Spread the dough evenly onto the prepared pan. Poke some holes in the bottom to prevent bubble formations.
6. Bake the crust for 11 minutes and remove from the oven. Place foil on the edges—return to the oven—for five to eight more minutes.
7. Let the crust cool completely.

For the Filling:
1. In a medium dish, combine the butter, ½ cup stevia, sour cream, cocoa powder, vanilla, and cream cheese.
2. Use the low-speed setting of a mixer to combine the mixture. Increase to a high-speed setting until all of the mixture is fluffy.
3. In a separate dish, whip the cream using high-speed (with clean beaters) until soft peaks are formed. Add one teaspoon of the vanilla extract and two teaspoons of the sweetener and whip until stiff peaks appear.
4. Blend in the whipped cream mix into the cream cheese mix. You are trying to combine the two mixtures while not removing any bubbles in the cream.
5. Scoop out the filling and smooth it out with a spoon. Chill the pie for a minimum of three hours.

Carbs: 10.6 g each (10 servings per recipe)

Chocolate Soufflé

Ingredients
1/3 cup sugar substitute (Lakanto Mont Fruit/Amazon)
1 tablespoon butter
5 ounces unsweetened chocolate
6 large egg whites
3 large egg yolks
The eggs work best at room temperature.

Instructions Preheat the oven to 375ºF. Use the butter to grease a soufflé dish.

1. Prepare a double boiler or a metal dish above a pan of boiling water to melt the chocolate. Stir the mix constantly. Remove the dish and whip in the yolks until the mix hardens. Set it aside.
2. With a pinch of salt, whisk the egg whites with an electric mixer on the highest setting. Gradually, blend in the sugar/Lakanto. Continue until you see stiff peaks.
3. Stir approximately one cup of the egg whites into the chocolate combination folding gently using a silicone spatula. Pour the mixture into the soufflé dish.
4. Bake approximately 20minutes. The center should still jiggle with the soufflé crusted and puffed on the top. Serve right away.

Note: To make the soufflé rise evenly, use your thumb to remove the batter from the top of the dish.

Carbs: 3.4 g (recipe is 4 servings)

Ginger Snap Cookies

Ingredients
¼ cup unsalted butter
1 large egg
2 cups almond flour
½ teaspoon ground cinnamon
1 cup sugar substitute/Erythritol (Swerve)
1 teaspoon vanilla extract
2 teaspoons ground ginger
¼ teaspoon each:
  - Salt
  - Ground cloves
  - Nutmeg

Instructions
1. Set the oven to 350°F.
2. Combine the dry ingredients in a small dish.
3. Combine the remainder components to the dry mixture, and mix using a hand blender/mixer. (The dough will be crumbly and stiff.)
4. Measure out the dough for each cookie and flatten with a fork or your fingers.
5. Bake for approximately 9 to 11 minutes or till they are browned.

Carbs: 1.21 g each (recipe 24 servings)

Indian Keto Coconut Bars

Ingredients
1 1/3 cups coconut milk - unsweetened
1 ¾ cups (4.6 ounces) unsweetened shredded coconut
3 ½ ounces ghee
1 teaspoon cardamon powder/ elaichi
4 tablespoons (1.4 ounces) Erythritol
10 to 20 saffron threads
Optional topping: Chopped almonds

Instructions
1. Combine the shredded coconut in a container with 1 ¼ cup of coconut milk and set it to the side for 30 minutes.
2. Add the saffron and Erythritol, along with the remainder of the milk, and mix until the sugar dissolves. Wait 30 minutes.
3. Melt the ghee in a wok on low and add the coconut mixture for five to seven minutes.
4. Add the cardamon/elaichi and cook an additional five minutes.
5. Butter a baking/barfi tray (6.3 square inches approximately). Spread the mixture into about ½-inch thickness and freeze for 2 to 2 ½ hours.
6. Cut into 15 pieces.

Carbs: 1.4 g each (recipe for 15 servings)

Macaroon Keto Bombs

Ingredients
½ cup shredded coconut
¼ cup almond flour
2 tablespoons sugar substitute (Swerve)
3 egg whites
1 tablespoon each:
- Coconut oil
- Vanilla extract

Instructions
1. Set the oven at 400°F.
2. In a small dish, mix the almond flour, coconut, and Swerve.
3. Use a small saucepan to melt the coconut oil. Add the vanilla extract.
4. *Note*: To mount the egg whites, place a medium dish in the freezer.
5. Add the oil to the flour mixture and blend well.
6. Place the egg whites in the cold dish and whip/whisk until stiff peaks are formed.
7. Blend the egg whites into the flour mixture. Spoon the mixture into a muffin cup or place them on a cookie sheet.
8. Bake the macaroons for eight minutes or until you see browned edges.
9. Cool the bombs before you attempt to remove them from the pan.

Carbs: 0.5 g each (recipe provides 10 servings)

Mocha Chia Pudding

Ingredients
2 tablespoons herbal coffee
1/3 cup each:
- Dry chia seeds
- Undiluted coconut cream

1 tablespoon each:
- Organic vanilla extract
- Swerve

2 tablespoons cacao nibs

Instructions
1. Simmer two cups of water with the herbal blend for 15 minutes until about one cup remains. Strain and blend with the cream, extract and swerve.
2. Toss in the cacao nibs and seeds, blending well.
3. Place in the serving containers and chill for about 30 minutes before time to serve.

Carbs: 2.25 each (recipe is for 2 servings)

Pumpkin Pudding

Ingredients
¼ cup pumpkin puree
1/3 cup granulated (Erythritol/Stevia)
½ teaspoon pumpkin pie spices
1 teaspoon xanthan gum
3 medium egg yolks
1 teaspoon vanilla extract
1 ½ cups whipping cream

Ingredients for the Cream Mixture
3 tablespoons granulated stevia
1 cup whipping cream
½ teaspoon vanilla extract

Instructions
1. Whisk the pumpkin spice, xanthan gum, sweetener, and salt in a dish until the texture is smooth. Add the yolks, puree, and vanilla extract to the mixture, and blend thoroughly.
2. Gradually blend the whipping cream until all of the cream is added.
3. Use medium heat and let the mixture come to a boil. Continue the process for approximately four to seven minutes until thickened.
4. Place the pudding in the refrigerator in a container. Stir every ten minutes.
5. Meanwhile, in a medium dish, use a mixer to whip the one cup of whipping cream resulting in stiff peaks. Add the vanilla and sweetener. Stir gently.
6. After the base pudding mixture has cooled, fold the whipped cream into the mix.
7. Scoop the pudding into small serving dishes and chill for a minimum of one to two hours.

Carbs: 9 g each (recipe for 6 servings)

Keto Zucchini Bread with Walnuts

Ingredients
½ cup olive oil
1 teaspoon vanilla extract
3 large eggs
2 ½ cups almond flour
½ teaspoon salt
1 ½ cups Erythritol
1 ½ teaspoons baking powder
¼ teaspoon ground ginger
1 teaspoon ground cinnamon
½ teaspoon nutmeg
1 cup grated zucchini
½ cup chopped walnuts

Instructions
1. Set the oven temperature to 350°F.
2. Whisk the eggs, vanilla, and oil. In another dish mix the salt, Erythritol, flour, ginger, nutmeg, cinnamon, and baking powder.
3. Use a paper towel or cheesecloth to remove water from the rinsed – grated zucchini. Whisk it into the mixture.
4. Add the dry ingredients slowly with a hand mixer.
5. Coat a 9x5 baking loaf pan with some non-stick spray, and add the bread mixture. Sprinkle the walnuts on top of the bread, and press in slightly with a spatula.
6. Bake 60 to 70 minutes until browned.

Carbs: 2.49 g each (16 servings recipe)

Conclusion

Thank for purchasing your personal copy of the *Ketogenic Recipes: Nutritious, Delicious And Simple Ketogenic Recipes To Spike Your Metabolism And Burn Stubborn Fat.* Let's hope it was informative and provided you with all of the tools you need to achieve your goals by using the well-chosen ketogenic recipes.

The next step is to gather your favorite recipes and head to the supermarket. Each of the recipes provided has been carefully planned, so the recipes are ready for you to enjoy without any guilt!

Finally, if you found this book useful in any way, a review on Amazon is always appreciated!

Index

Chapter 1: Breakfast Delights

- Deviled Eggs
- Fisherman's Eggs
- Fried Eggs with Pork and Kale
- Frittata with Cheese and Tomatoes
- Italian Egg Bake
- Mock 'Mc Griddle' Casserole
- Omelet Wrap with Avocado & Salmon
- Sausage Patties
- Sausage—Feta—Spinach Omelet
- Scrambled Eggs and Bacon
- Sesame Buns
- Shakshuka
- **Spinach Alfredo & Avocado Eggs**

The Sweeter Side of Breakfast
- Blueberry Ricotta Pancakes
- Brownie Muffins
- Coconut Chia Bars
- Ham and Apple Flatbread

Chapter 2: Beef Choices

- Korean BBQ Keto Bowl
- Mississippi Roast – Slow Cooker
- Steak with Mushroom Port Sauce
- Steak-Lovers Slow-Cooked Chili
- Ground Beef Recipes
- Ground Beef Stir Fry
- Nachos or Tacos
- Spaghetti Squash Lasagna
- Hamburger Stroganoff
- Sweet and Sour Meatballs

Chapter 3: Chicken Duck and Turkey Choices

- Chicken—Broccoli—Zucchini Boats
- Chicken Smothered in Creamy Onion Sauce
- Chicken Stuffed Avocado—Cajun Style
- Creamy Chicken Casserole
- Roasted Chicken
- Turducken
- Roasted Duck
- Skillet Style Sausage and Cabbage Melt

Chapter 4: Pork Choices

- Keto Rack of Ribs
- Spaghetti Squash Meatballs
- Squash and Sausage Casserole
- Sunflower Pork & Butter Kabobs
- Tenderloin Stuffed Keto Style
- Thai Pork Salad with Kelp Noodles

Chapter 5: Seafood Recipes

- Baked Salmon
- Coconut Shrimp
- Rockfish with Creamy Ginger Avocado Dressing
- Sardine Fritters

Tuna Avocado Melt

Chapter 6: Salads – Sides – Sauces – Soups - and Snacks
Salads

- Asparagus and Radish Salad
- Avocado and Bacon Salad
- Bistro Steak Salad with Horseradish Dressing
- Bok-Choy Salad – Oven-Baked
- Mixed Green Spring Salad
- Zucchini and Walnut Salad

Veggies and Sides
- Deep-Fat Fried Spicy Brussels Sprouts
- Cauliflower Hash Browns
- Cauliflower Rice
- Keto Cole Slaw
- Southern Fried Cabbage
- Spaghetti Squash
- Stuffed Green Peppers – Keto Style

Sauces
- Low-Carb Mayonnaise

Soups
- Beef Bone Broth
- Cauliflower Soup with Crumbled Pancetta
- Chicken and Chili Soup - Crock Pot
- Chorizo and Chicken Soup - Crock Pot

Snacks
- Bacon Wrapped Scallops
- Beef and Bacon Rolls
- Mini Eggplant Pizza - Keto
- Pizza Base
- Raw Spiraled Zucchini Noodles with Tomatoes and Pesto
- Zucchini and Goat Cheese Wraps

Chapter 7: Desserts

- Brownie Cheesecake
- No-Bake Cashew Coconut Bars
- Cheesecake Lemon Moose
- Chocolate Silk Pie
- Chocolate Soufflé
- Ginger Snap Cookies
- Indian Keto Coconut Bars
- Macaroon Keto Bombs
- Mocha Chia Pudding
- Pumpkin Pudding
- Zucchini Bread with Walnuts